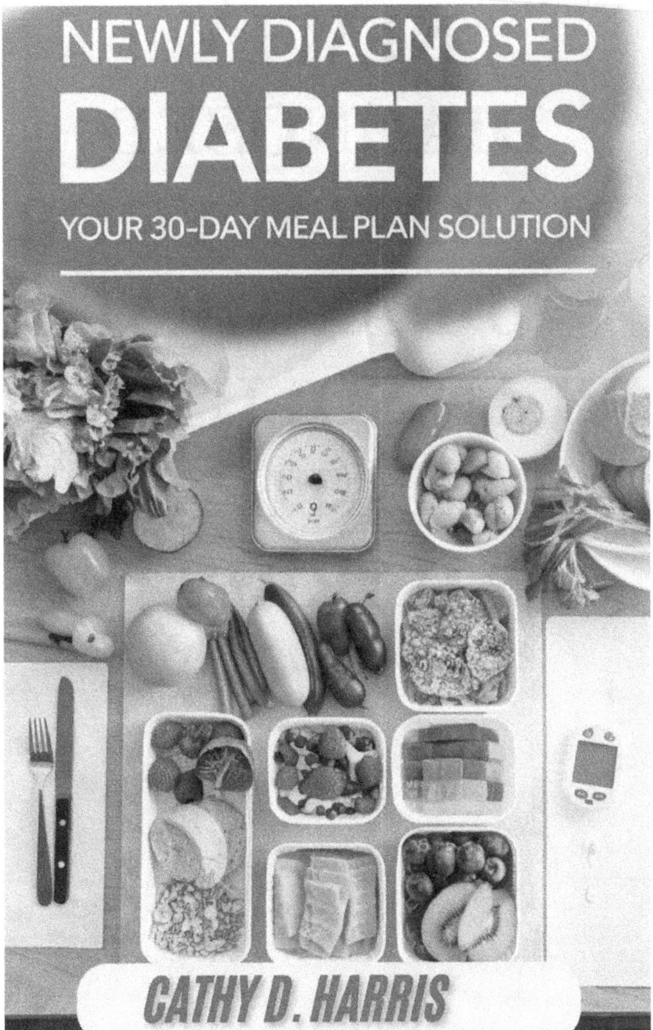

NEWLY DIAGNOSED
DIABETES

YOUR 30-DAY MEAL PLAN SOLUTION

CATHY D. HARRIS

NEWLY DIAGNOSED DIABETES: YOUR 30-DAY MEAL PLAN SOLUTION BY CATHY D. HARRIS

COPYRIGHT

DISCLAIMER

The information provided in this book is for general informational and educational purposes only. It is not intended as, nor should it be considered, a substitute for professional advice, diagnosis, or treatment. The author is not a licensed therapist, counselor, or medical professional. Readers should consult a qualified professional for any matters regarding their mental, emotional, or physical health.

The strategies, suggestions, and techniques outlined in this book are based on the author's personal experiences and research. Results may vary, and the reader's use of the information provided is at their own risk. The author and publisher assume no responsibility or liability for any consequences, injuries, or damages resulting from the use of the information contained in this book.

By reading this book, you agree to hold the author and publisher harmless from any claims, actions, or demands arising from your use of the information provided herein.

ABOUT THE AUTHOR

Cathy D. Harris is a passionate advocate for personal growth and improvement. With a deep belief in the power of mindset and intentional living, Cathy has dedicated her life to helping others break free from limiting beliefs and realize their full potential. Her journey into the world of self-help began with her own struggles to overcome self-doubt and fear. Through years of learning, practice, and perseverance,

Cathy transformed her life and now shares her insights with others.

Cathy's writing is grounded in her personal experiences and her commitment to making complex ideas accessible and practical for everyone. She believes that anyone can create a life they love with the right tools and mindset, and her work is a testament to this philosophy.

In addition to her writing, Cathy is a sought-after speaker and coach, known for her relatable approach and down-to-earth advice. She connects with her audience on a personal level, encouraging them to take actionable steps toward lasting change.

When she's not writing or speaking, Cathy enjoys spending time in nature, practicing mindfulness, and continuously exploring new ways to grow and evolve. She lives by the mantra that every day is an opportunity to be better, do better, and live better.

Cathy D. Harris is excited to share her journey with you and hopes that her book will inspire you to unleash your potential and create the life you've always dreamed of.

TABLE OF CONTENTS

INTRODUCTION: NEWLY DIAGNOSED DIABETES

If you've just found out you have diabetes, it might seem scary. But, with the right diet and lifestyle, you can manage it well. This guide will help you feel more in control of your health.

This guide has a special 30-day meal plan for people with new diabetes. It teaches you how to keep your blood sugar right with food, portion sizes, and lifestyle changes. It's a step towards a healthier future.

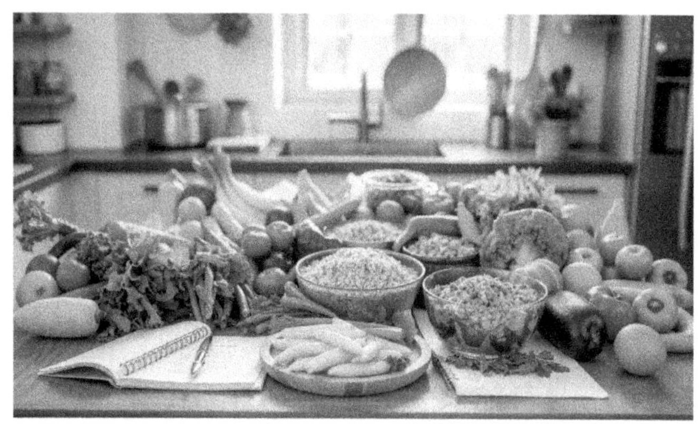

A vibrant kitchen scene featuring a beautifully arranged table with a variety of healthy foods suited for a diabetes meal plan, including colorful vegetables, whole grains, lean proteins, and fresh fruits, all presented in an inviting manner, soft natural lighting highlighting the freshness of the ingredients, surrounded by cooking utensils and a meal plan notebook laid open nearby, creating a warm and encouraging atmosphere for healthy eating.

Key Takeaways

- Understand the common symptoms and initial steps

to take after a diabetes diagnosis.

- Learn about the different types of diabetes and the role of blood sugar monitoring.

- Discover the importance of structured meal planning for effective diabetes management.

- Explore essential kitchen tools and ingredients for your diabetic meal prep.

- Master carbohydrate counting and portion

control strategies to stabilize blood sugar levels.

Understanding Your New Diabetes Diagnosis

Getting a diabetes diagnosis can feel scary. But knowing what it is is the first step to managing it. Diabetes is when your body can't control blood sugar levels. This can lead to serious health problems.

As you start this new journey, let's look at symptoms, types of diabetes, and why checking blood sugar is important.

Common Symptoms and Initial Steps

Diabetes symptoms include being very thirsty, needing to pee a lot, losing weight without trying, feeling tired, and blurry vision. If you notice these, see a doctor right away. They will do tests to see if you have diabetes and what to do next.

Types of Diabetes Explained

- *Type 1 Diabetes:* This happens when your body attacks and destroys insulin-making cells in your pancreas. You then don't make insulin anymore.

- *Type 2 Diabetes:* This is when your body doesn't use insulin well. This makes your blood sugar levels too high.

- *Gestational Diabetes:* This type happens during pregnancy. It usually goes away after the baby is born. But it can raise your risk of getting type 2 diabetes later.

The Role of Blood Sugar Monitoring

Checking your blood sugar often is key to managing diabetes. It shows how your body reacts to food, exercise, and medicine. This info helps you and your doctor make a plan to keep your blood sugar healthy.

This plan helps avoid serious problems like insulin resistance and blood sugar control.

Remember, diabetes education is crucial. It helps you understand your condition and take charge of your health. By working with your doctor, you can manage your diabetes and stay healthy.

The Importance of Structured Meal Planning for Diabetes Management

Proper meal planning is key for managing diabetes and staying healthy. It helps control blood sugar, lowers risk of problems, and boosts life quality.

Structured meal planning helps keep blood sugar stable. It makes it easier to eat the right foods. This keeps blood sugar levels in check, avoiding big swings.

It also boosts overall health and happiness. Eating foods rich in nutrients helps get all needed vitamins and minerals. This improves energy and reduces health risks.

It also helps with weight management, which is very important for diabetics. Eating the right amount of food helps keep a healthy weight. This reduces body strain and health risks.

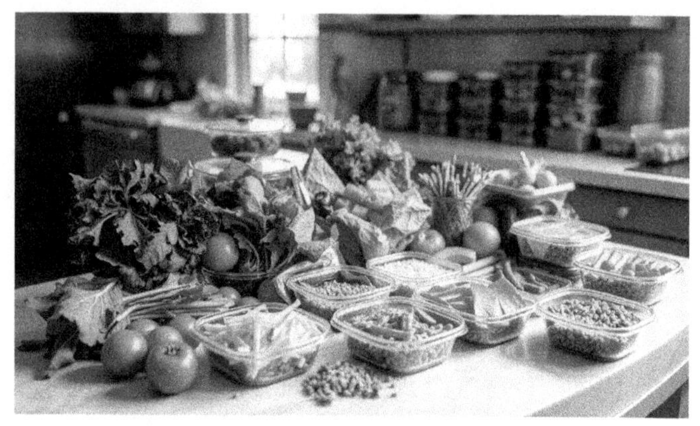

A vibrant kitchen table filled with fresh, colorful ingredients for meal prep, including leafy greens, lean proteins, whole grains, and a variety of vegetables; organized meal containers in the background; a serene atmosphere with natural light streaming in through a window, showcasing a healthy lifestyle and mindful eating choices.

In short, meal planning is very important for diabetes management. It helps control blood sugar, keeps health good, and lowers risk of problems. With good planning, diabetics can live a full and balanced life.

Essential Kitchen Tools and Ingredients for Your Diabetic Meal Prep

Starting a diabetic lifestyle means changing how you eat and setting up your kitchen right. You need the right tools and ingredients to plan and make meals well. We'll look at the kitchen gear, pantry items, and shopping tips for tasty, healthy meals that help your health.

Must-Have Kitchen Equipment

Having the right kitchen tools is key for a diabetic lifestyle. Here are some must-haves:

- Digital food scale: It's important for healthy meal planning and dietary guidelines.
- Nonstick cookware: It helps you cook without extra oils and fats, making meals better for diabetes.
- Slow cooker: It's great for making tasty, healthy meals with little effort, perfect for busy days.

- Blender or food processor: It's good for making smoothies, dips, and sauces that fit into a diabetic lifestyle.

Diabetes-Friendly Pantry Staples

Having the right pantry items is crucial for a healthy meal planning routine. Here are some dietary guidelines-approved items:

1. Whole grains (quinoa, brown rice, oats)
2. Lean proteins (chicken, fish, tofu, legumes)
3. Healthy fats (olive oil, avocado, nuts, seeds)
4. Fresh or frozen vegetables and fruits
5. Low-sugar condiments and spices

Smart Shopping Guidelines

Shopping smart is key when you're watching your diet. Here are some tips:

- Read nutrition labels well, looking at carbs, fiber, and sugar.
- Choose whole, less processed foods when you can.
- Look for fresh foods on the store's edges.
- Plan your meals and list what you need to avoid buying things that don't fit your dietary guidelines.

With the right kitchen tools and pantry items, you can make tasty, healthy meals. These meals will help you stay healthy and feel good.

Carbohydrate Counting: Your New Best Friend

Getting used to diabetes means learning to count carbs. This skill helps you control your blood sugar and manage your diabetes.

Carbs are in foods like bread, pasta, fruits, and sweets. They affect your blood sugar. By tracking carbs, you can avoid big blood sugar jumps and keep it stable.

Carb Counting Essentials

Here are some tips to start carb counting:

- Get a carb-counting app or food guide. These help you know the carbs in different foods.

- Look at nutrition labels for carbs. This helps you pick the right food amounts.

- Learn about common carb foods and their carb counts. This helps you guess carbs even without labels.

Carb counting takes time to get good at. Be patient and ask for help from your doctor or dietitian. With effort, you'll get better at it. This will help you control your blood sugar and manage your diabetes better.

"Carb counting is the foundation for achieving

dietary guidelines and maintaining healthy blood sugar levels."

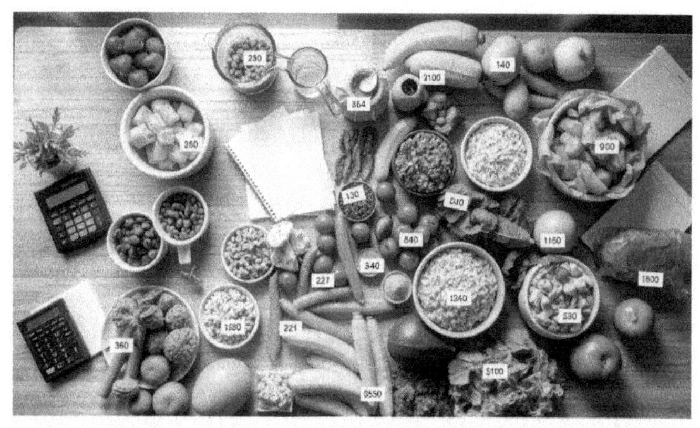

A visually appealing table filled with various foods, each item labeled with its carbohydrate count. Include a variety of colorful fruits, vegetables, grains, and proteins arranged neatly. Surround the table with measuring cups, a calculator, and a notepad for tracking carbs. Soft natural light illuminates the scene to create a warm, inviting atmosphere.

Portion Control Strategies for Blood Sugar Management

Keeping the right portion sizes is key for managing diabetes. It helps keep blood sugar levels healthy. There are simple ways to make sure you eat the right amount at each meal.

Using the Plate Method

The plate method is a visual tool for balanced meals. Here's how it works:

- Divide your plate into three sections. One-half for non-starchy veggies, one-quarter for lean protein, and one-quarter for complex carbs.

- This helps control carb intake and keeps blood sugar stable.

- It also encourages eating more fiber-rich, nutrient-dense foods for better health.

Measuring Portions Without Tools

You can guess portion sizes without measuring cups or a food scale. Here are some tips:

1. *Palm of your hand:* Use your palm to measure protein like meat, fish, or poultry.
2. *Cupped hand:* A cupped handful is good for carbs like rice, pasta, or cereal.
3. *Thumb tip:* The tip of your thumb is about a teaspoon. It's useful for oils, nut butters, and healthy fats.

Mastering these portion control strategies helps you manage

diabetes. It keeps your blood sugar stable all day.

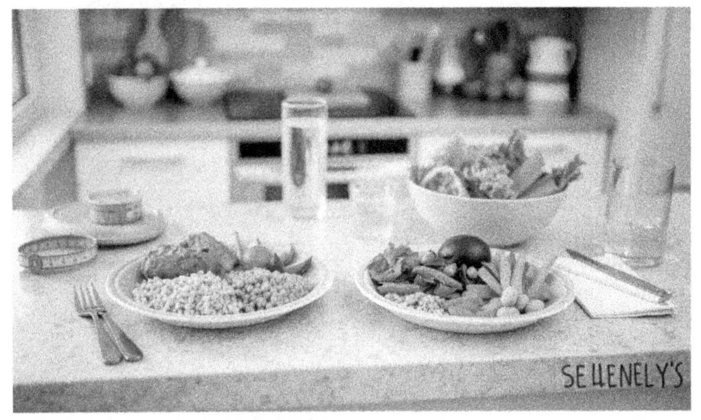

A visually appealing kitchen countertop featuring a balanced meal divided into controlled portions using colorful plates and bowls. Include a variety of healthy foods like lean proteins, whole grains, and fresh vegetables arranged in moderate amounts. Incorporate measuring tools like a scale or measuring cups nearby, along with a food diary and a glass of water. The atmosphere should be bright and inviting, promoting a sense of health and wellness.

Newly Diagnosed Diabetes: Your 30-Day Meal Plan Solution

Starting a new life with diabetes can feel scary. But, with the right help, it's easier. This 30-day meal plan is made for new diabetes patients. It helps keep blood sugar levels stable and keeps you healthy.

This plan focuses on foods that are good for you. It includes meals and snacks that are full of nutrients. Eating whole, unprocessed foods helps you manage diabetes better. It also helps you live a healthier life.

The main parts of this meal plan are:

- Recipes made just for diabetes patients to control blood sugar.
- Meals with complex carbs, lean proteins, and healthy fats for a full feeling.
- Portions that help you stay at a healthy weight and control blood sugar.
- Plans that fit different diets and lifestyles, making it easy to follow.

By using this 30-day meal plan, you learn how to manage diabetes. You also start good habits that last longer than 30 days. Start your journey to better diabetes management and health today.

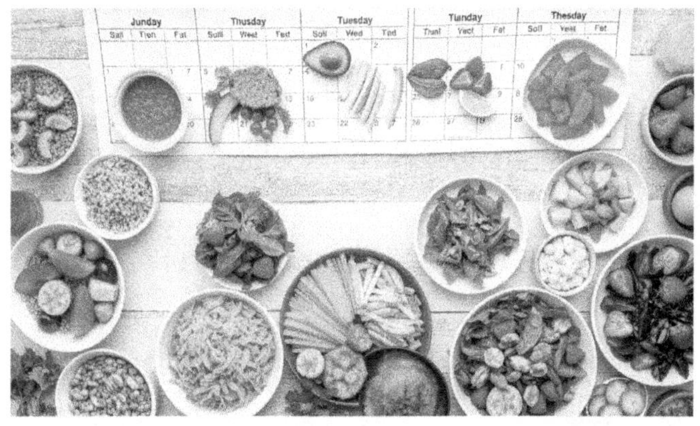

A vibrant table set with a variety of colorful, healthy

dishes, showcasing a 30-day meal plan for diabetes management. Include whole grains, fresh fruits, lean proteins, leafy greens, and nuts. The background features a calendar with each day visually represented by different meals and ingredients, all arranged in an appetizing and inviting manner. Emphasize balance and nutrition with bright colors and appealing presentation.

"The key to successful diabetes management is found in the daily choices we make, and this 30-day meal plan solution provides the framework to make those choices with confidence."

Breakfast Ideas That Won't Spike Blood Sugar

Keeping blood sugar stable is key for diabetes management. Breakfast is especially important. Try these low-carb recipes for energy without blood sugar spikes.

Quick Morning Meals

- Scrambled eggs with spinach and a side of avocado
- *Protein-packed yogurt parfait with berries and nuts*
- Veggie-filled omelet with a sprinkle of cheese

Weekend Breakfast Options

1. Baked oatmeal with almond milk, cinnamon, and blueberries
2. Crustless quiche loaded with low-carb veggies
3. *Savory breakfast burrito wrapped in a lettuce leaf*

For diabetes-friendly breakfasts, choose low-carb recipes, blood sugar control, and diabetes management. Lean proteins, healthy fats, and fiber-rich foods are best. They give you steady energy and stable glucose levels.

"Breakfast is the most important meal of the day, especially for those managing diabetes. These recipes will help you enjoy a satisfying, blood sugar-friendly start to your morning."

Lunch and Dinner Combinations for Stable Glucose Levels

Keeping blood sugar steady is key for people with diabetes. Lunch and dinner should have lean proteins, healthy fats, and complex carbs. This helps keep blood sugar healthy and supports *healthy meal planning* and *blood sugar control.*

Use the plate method to plan your meals. Start with lean protein like grilled chicken or tofu. Then, add non-starchy veggies like leafy greens or broccoli. Finish with a small portion of a *low-carb recipe* like brown rice or a small baked potato.

Lunch Idea	Dinner Idea
Chicken Cobb Salad with Avocado and Hard Boiled Egg	Grilled Salmon with Roasted Asparagus and Quinoa

Tuna Lettuce Wraps with Cucumber and Tomato	Baked Chicken Breast with Roasted Brussels Sprouts and Sweet Potato
Beef and Vegetable Stir-Fry with	Baked Cod with Sautéed Spinach and Cauliflower Rice

Brown Rice	

For diabetes, eat foods that are rich in nutrients but low in sugar. These balanced meals help manage diabetes and improve health.

Smart Snacking Strategies for Diabetics

Keeping your blood sugar stable is key for managing diabetes. Smart snacking is a big help. It lets you eat between meals and keep your blood sugar in check.

Between-Meal Blood Sugar Control

Choosing the right snacks is very important. Look for snacks low in carbs and high in fiber, protein, or healthy fats. Good choices are:

- Sliced vegetables with hummus or Greek yogurt
- Handful of nuts or seeds
- Hard-boiled eggs

- Cottage cheese with berries

These snacks help keep your blood sugar steady. They stop big spikes or drops.

Emergency Snack Options

Having emergency snacks ready is also key. They give you quick energy or stop blood sugar dips. Some good emergency snacks are:

1. Individual packets of nut butter or cheese crisps

2. Low-sugar granola bars or protein bars

3. Fresh fruit, such as apples, bananas, or grapes

These snacks are quick and easy to use. They help control your blood sugar when you need it.

Adding these smart snacking tips to your day helps a lot with diabetes management. It keeps your blood sugar stable all day.

Eating Out While Managing Diabetes

Living with diabetes makes eating out hard. But, with smart planning, you can still enjoy meals. Here are tips to help you stay on track with your diabetic lifestyle and diabetes management when eating out.

Scan the Menu Ahead of Time

Look at the menu online before you go. This helps you find

diabetes-friendly options. Choose meals with lean proteins, veggies, and complex carbs.

Ask Questions and Customize Orders

Talk to your server about what you need. Ask for changes like grilled instead of fried. Most places will make these changes to make your meal better.

Be Mindful of Portion Sizes

Watch how much you eat. Use the "plate method" to guide you. Fill half with veggies, a quarter with protein, and a quarter with carbs. Don't eat everything on your plate.

Manage Carbohydrates Wisely

Be careful of carbs in sauces and dressings. Keep track of carbs to adjust your insulin. This helps keep your blood sugar stable.

Eating out with diabetes needs planning and attention. But, with these tips, you can enjoy meals out. You won't have to give up your diabetic lifestyle or diabetes management.

Exercise and Meal Timing: Creating the Perfect Balance

Living with diabetes means finding the right balance between exercise and meal timing. This balance helps keep your blood sugar levels healthy.

Eating the right foods before and after working out is key to managing your diabetes management and reaching your fitness goals.

Pre-Workout Nutrition

Before you start exercising, fuel your body with the right mix of nutrients. Look for a snack or small meal with complex carbs, lean protein, and healthy fats. This mix helps keep your blood sugar control steady and gives you energy for your workout.

Good pre-workout snacks for diabetics include:

- Greek yogurt with berries and a sprinkle of nuts
- Whole-grain toast with avocado and a hard-boiled egg
- A small apple with a tablespoon of nut butter

Post-Exercise Meal Planning

After working out, it's crucial to refuel with the right nutrients.

A balanced meal with complex carbs, lean protein, and healthy fats helps regulate your blood sugar. It also supports muscle recovery. Some good post-workout meals are:

1. Grilled chicken breast with roasted sweet potatoes and steamed broccoli
2. Quinoa and black bean salad with diced tomatoes and olive oil
3. Salmon filet with roasted Brussels sprouts and brown rice

Remember, everyone's body is different. Pay attention to how you react to different exercises and foods. Talk to your healthcare team to create a plan that's just right for you.

"Proper nutrition before and after exercise can make a significant difference in managing your diabetes and achieving your fitness goals."

Monitoring and Adjusting Your Meal Plan

Managing diabetes is a dynamic process. Your meal plan needs regular checks and tweaks. This ensures you keep your blood sugar in check and manage your diabetes well.

By watching how your body reacts to the 30-day meal plan, you can make smart changes. These changes help you fine-tune your diet for better results.

The secret to good diabetes management is adapting and making your meal plan your own. Here are some important steps to follow:

1. Keep track of your blood sugar levels every day. Write down your readings and look for any patterns.

2. See how your body reacts to different foods and how they mix together. Find out which foods keep your blood sugar stable.

3. Change your carbohydrate intake and portion sizes if needed. This helps keep your blood sugar in balance.

4. Try new healthy meals and add more diabetes-friendly ingredients to your plan.

5. Meet with your healthcare team often. They can help you adjust your meal plan or medication as needed.

Remember, managing diabetes is not a one-size-fits-all deal.

By watching your progress and making changes, you can keep your meal plan working for you.

"The key to successful diabetes management is your ability to adapt and personalize your meal plan."

Management

choosing breakfasts that are rich in protein and healthy fats, while low in refined carbs, can help maintain stable blood sugar levels throughout the morning. These meal options offer a balanced combination of nutrients that will not only keep you feeling full but also provide steady energy to start your day without the risk of blood sugar spikes.

Lunch Ideas for Balanced Energy

Lunch is a great opportunity to refuel with a nutritious meal that keeps your blood sugar levels in check. Focus on meals that combine lean protein, healthy fats, and high-fiber vegetables. Here are some ideas:

Grilled chicken salad with leafy greens, cherry tomatoes, and a light olive oil dressing

Lentil soup with a side of whole-grain crackers

Turkey and avocado lettuce wrap with a side of cucumber slices

Quinoa bowl with roasted vegetables, chickpeas, and a drizzle of tahini dressing

These meals are rich in fiber, which helps slow down sugar absorption, stabilizing blood sugar levels while keeping you satisfied.

Dinner Ideas for Blood Sugar Control

Dinner should be filling but not overwhelming, allowing you to wind down while still managing blood sugar. Focus on lean proteins and plenty of vegetables:

Grilled salmon with roasted Brussels sprouts and quinoa

Stir-fried tofu with broccoli, bell peppers, and brown rice

Chicken and vegetable skewers with a side of cauliflower rice

Baked cod with sweet potato and steamed green beans

These meals provide healthy fats and fiber, ensuring your evening meal supports your overall diabetes management.

Snack Ideas That Support Stable Blood Sugar

Snacks are important for maintaining energy and preventing dips in blood sugar. Choose snacks that are balanced and contain a mix of protein, fiber, and healthy fats:

Apple slices with almond butter

Greek yogurt with a sprinkle of chia seeds

Cottage cheese with cucumber and cherry tomatoes

Carrot sticks with hummus

These snacks are not only low in sugar but also packed with nutrients that support stable blood sugar levels.

By following these meal ideas and incorporating the 30-day meal plan into your routine, you can take control of your diabetes management and set yourself up for success. With the right foods and strategies, you'll be able to maintain balanced blood sugar levels and live a healthier, more energized life.

Conclusion

Starting your journey with diabetes? This 30-day meal plan is a great start. It helps you manage your diabetes well. You'll learn about meal planning, counting carbs, and controlling portions.

This guide also shows you how to shop and cook healthy meals. You'll find tasty breakfasts, lunches, dinners, and snacks. It's all about eating right for your needs.

Managing diabetes takes time and effort. But with the right tools and a good plan, you can do it. Keep an eye on your blood sugar, exercise often, and stick to your meal plan. You'll feel better and more in control.